THE ONE-MINUTE GRATITUDE JOURNAL FOR WOMEN

A JOURNAL FOR SELF-CARE AND HAPPINESS

This Journal belongs to

_____

Gratitude

Gratitude is a feeling of appreciation for what one has. It is a feeling of thankfulness for the blessings we have received. Cultivating an attitude of gratitude yields many benefits: physical, mental and spiritual. Feeling gratitude in the present moment makes you happier and more relaxed, and improves your overall health and well-being.

Write down three to five things that you are grateful for each day. You will not only feel good as you write them down, but you will experience gratitude during the day as well. A person experiencing gratitude feels a sense of joy and abundance in their life. They also feel more connected with other people and have increased energy.

It should come as no surprise to learn that stress amongst women is very common. The act of writing down what you are grateful for, can help relieve stress and anxiety.

Remember, it's your journal, so you can list whatever you like, no matter how big or small it may be, as long as it brings pleasure to your life.

There are pages in this journal where you can just draw something. If you don't feel like drawing anything, simply paste a beautiful picture onto this page. Our minds react better to imagery and this is a great way to feel gratitude and appreciation.

Gratitude makes us more optimistic and compassionate. True happiness lies within us. By keeping a record of your gratitude in a journal, you will store positive energy, gain clarity in your life, and have greater control of your thoughts and emotions.

Each day, write down three to five things that you are grateful for in this journal and turn your ordinary moments into blessings.

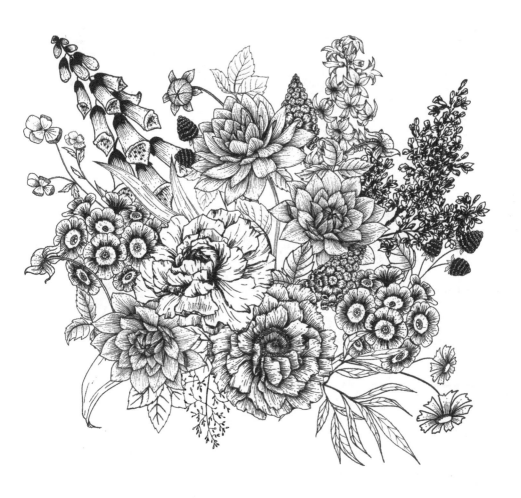

Day: _____ *Date:* ____/____/____

Today I am *Grateful* for _____

_____

_____

_____

_____

_____

_____

Happiness depends upon ourselves.
~ *Aristotle*

Day: _____ *Date:* ____/____/____

Today I am *Grateful* for _____

_____

_____

_____

_____

_____

Day: _____ *Date:* _____ / _____ / _____

Today I am *Grateful* for _____

_____

_____

_____

_____

_____

_____

No act of kindness, no matter how small, is ever wasted.
~ *Aesop*

Day: _____ *Date:* _____ / _____ / _____

Today I am *Grateful* for _____

_____

_____

_____

_____

_____

Day: _____ *Date:* _____ / _____ / _____

Today I am *Grateful* for _____

_____

_____

_____

_____

_____

_____

Success is sweet and sweeter if long delayed and gotten through
many struggles and defeats. ~ *Amos Bronson Alcott*

Day: _____ *Date:* _____ / _____ / _____

Today I am *Grateful* for _____

_____

_____

_____

_____

_____

_____

Day: _____ *Date:* ____/____/____

Today I am *Grateful* for _____

_____

_____

_____

_____

_____

Happiness is a choice that requires effort at times.
~ *Aeschylus*

Day: _____ *Date:* ____/____/____

Today I am *Grateful* for _____

_____

_____

_____

_____

_____

Day: _____ *Date:* ____ / ____ / ____

Today I am *Grateful* for

_____

_____

_____

_____

_____

_____

The energy of the mind is the essence of life.
~ *Aristotle*

Day: _____ *Date:* ____ / ____ / ____

Today I am *Grateful* for

_____

_____

_____

_____

_____

_____

Day: _____ *Date:* _____ / _____ / _____

Today I am *Grateful* for _____

_____

_____

_____

_____

_____

To the artist there is never anything ugly in nature.
~ *Auguste Rodin*

Day: _____ *Date:* _____ / _____ / _____

Today I am *Grateful* for _____

_____

_____

_____

_____

_____

Day: _____ *Date:* _____ / _____ / _____

Today I am *Grateful* for _____

_____

_____

_____

_____

_____

Happiness is a virtue, not its reward.
~ *Baruch Spinoza*

Day: _____ *Date:* _____ / _____ / _____

Today I am *Grateful* for _____

_____

_____

_____

_____

Day: _____ *Date:* ____ / ____ / ____

Today I am *Grateful* for _____

_____

_____

_____

_____

_____

It is not knowledge, but the act of learning, not possession
but the act of getting there, which grants the greatest enjoyment.
~ Carl Friedrich

Day: _____ *Date:* ____ / ____ / ____

Today I am *Grateful* for _____

_____

_____

_____

_____

_____

Day: _____ *Date:* ____ / ____ / ____

Today I am *Grateful* for _____

_____

_____

_____

_____

_____

Wherever you go, go with all your heart.
~ *Confucius*

Day: _____ *Date:* ____ / ____ / ____

Today I am *Grateful* for _____

_____

_____

_____

_____

_____

Day: _____ *Date:* ____ / ____ / ____

Today I am *Grateful* for _____

_____

_____

_____

_____

_____

_____

I hear and I forget. I see and I remember. I do and I understand.
~ Confucius

Day: _____ *Date:* ____ / ____ / ____

Today I am *Grateful* for _____

_____

_____

_____

_____

_____

_____

Day: _____ *Date:* ____ / ____ / ____

Today I am *Grateful* for _____

_____

_____

_____

_____

_____

Good means not merely not to do wrong, but rather not to desire
to do wrong. ~ *Democritus*

Day: _____ *Date:* ____ / ____ / ____

Today I am *Grateful* for _____

_____

_____

_____

_____

_____

Day: _____ *Date:* ____ / ____ / ____

Today I am *Grateful* for _____

_____

_____

_____

_____

_____

There are two ways of spreading light: to be the candle or
the mirror that reflects it. ~ *Edith Wharton*

Day: _____ *Date:* ____ / ____ / ____

Today I am *Grateful* for _____

_____

_____

_____

_____

_____

Day: _____ *Date:* ____/____/____

Today I am *Grateful* for _____

_____

_____

_____

_____

_____

True originality consists not in a new manner but in a
new vision. ~ *Edith Wharton*

Day: _____ *Date:* ____/____/____

Today I am *Grateful* for _____

_____

_____

_____

_____

_____

Day: _____ *Date:* _____ / _____ / _____

Today I am *Grateful* for _____

_____

_____

_____

_____

_____

_____

Make it your habit not to be critical about small things.
~ *Edward Everett Hale*

Day: _____ *Date:* _____ / _____ / _____

Today I am *Grateful* for _____

_____

_____

_____

_____

_____

Draw something

Day: _____ *Date:* _____ / _____ / _____

Today I am *Grateful* for _____

_____

_____

_____

_____

_____

_____

Positive anything is better than negative nothing.
~ *Elbert Hubbard*

Day: _____ *Date:* _____ / _____ / _____

Today I am *Grateful* for _____

_____

_____

_____

_____

_____

Day: _____ *Date:* _____ / _____ / _____

Today I am *Grateful* for _____

_____

_____

_____

_____

_____

Find ecstasy in life; the mere sense of living is joy enough.
~ *Emily Dickinson*

Day: _____ *Date:* _____ / _____ / _____

Today I am *Grateful* for _____

_____

_____

_____

_____

_____

Day: _____ *Date:* _____ / _____ / _____

Today I am *Grateful* for _____

_____

_____

_____

_____

_____

To live is so startling it leaves little time for anything else.
~ *Emily Dickinson*

Day: _____ *Date:* _____ / _____ / _____

Today I am *Grateful* for _____

_____

_____

_____

_____

_____

Day: _____ *Date:* _____ / _____ / _____

Today I am *Grateful* for _____

_____

_____

_____

_____

_____

There is only one way to happiness and that is to cease worrying
about things which are beyond the power of our will. ~ *Epictetus*

Day: _____ *Date:* _____ / _____ / _____

Today I am *Grateful* for _____

_____

_____

_____

_____

_____

Day: _____ *Date:* ____ / ____ / ____

Today I am *Grateful* for _____

_____

_____

_____

_____

_____

Events will take their course, it is no good of being angry at them;
he is happiest who wisely turns them to the best account. ~ *Euripides*

Day: _____ *Date:* ____ / ____ / ____

Today I am *Grateful* for _____

_____

_____

_____

_____

_____

Day: _____ *Date:* ____/____/____

Today I am *Grateful* for _____

_____

_____

_____

_____

_____

We love life, not because we are used to living but because we are
used to loving. ~ *Friedrich Nietzsche*

Day: _____ *Date:* ____/____/____

Today I am *Grateful* for _____

_____

_____

_____

_____

_____

Day: _____ *Date:* _____ / _____ / _____

Today I am *Grateful* for _____

_____

_____

_____

_____

_____

One must still have chaos in oneself to be able to give birth
to a dancing star. ~ *Friedrich Nietzsche*

Day: _____ *Date:* _____ / _____ / _____

Today I am *Grateful* for _____

_____

_____

_____

_____

_____

Day: _____ *Date:* _____ / _____ / _____

Today I am *Grateful* for _____

_____

_____

_____

_____

_____

Grace is the beauty of form under the influence of freedom.
~ *Friedrich Schiller*

Day: _____ *Date:* _____ / _____ / _____

Today I am *Grateful* for _____

_____

_____

_____

_____

_____

Day: _____ *Date:* ____ / ____ / ____

Today I am *Grateful* for _____

_____

_____

_____

_____

_____

_____

Blessed is the influence of one true, loving human soul on another.
~ *George Eliot*

Day: _____ *Date:* ____ / ____ / ____

Today I am *Grateful* for _____

_____

_____

_____

_____

_____

Day: _____ *Date:* ____ / ____ / ____

Today I am *Grateful* for _____

_____

_____

_____

_____

_____

A single grateful thought toward heaven is the most perfect prayer.
~ *Gotthold Ephraim Lessing*

Day: _____ *Date:* ____ / ____ / ____

Today I am *Grateful* for _____

_____

_____

_____

_____

_____

Day: _____ *Date:* _____ / _____ / _____

Today I am *Grateful* for _____

_____

_____

_____

_____

_____

Never give up, for that is just the place and time that the tide
will turn. ~ *Harriet Beecher Stowe*

Day: _____ *Date:* _____ / _____ / _____

Today I am *Grateful* for _____

_____

_____

_____

_____

_____

Day: _____ *Date:* ____ / ____ / ____

Today I am *Grateful* for _____

_____

_____

_____

_____

_____

_____

When words leave off, music begins.
~ Heinrich Heine

Day: _____ *Date:* ____ / ____ / ____

Today I am *Grateful* for _____

_____

_____

_____

_____

_____

_____

Day: _____ *Date:* ____ / ____ / ____

Today I am *Grateful* for _____

_____

_____

_____

_____

_____

A thousand words will not leave so deep an impression as
one deed. ~ *Henrik Ibsen*

Day: _____ *Date:* ____ / ____ / ____

Today I am *Grateful* for _____

_____

_____

_____

_____

_____

Day: _____ *Date:* ____ / ____ / ____

Today I am *Grateful* for _____

_____

_____

_____

_____

_____

All experience is an arch, to build upon.
~ *Henry Adams*

Day: _____ *Date:* ____ / ____ / ____

Today I am *Grateful* for _____

_____

_____

_____

_____

_____

Draw something

Day: _____ *Date:* ____ / ____ / ____

Today I am *Grateful* for _____

_____

_____

_____

_____

_____

_____

Courtesies of a small and trivial character are the ones which
strike deepest in the grateful and appreciating heart. ~ *Henry Clay*

Day: _____ *Date:* ____ / ____ / ____

Today I am *Grateful* for _____

_____

_____

_____

_____

_____

Day: _____ *Date:* ____ / ____ / ____

Today I am *Grateful* for _____

_____

_____

_____

_____

_____

This world is but a canvas to our imagination.
~ *Henry David Thoreau*

Day: _____ *Date:* ____ / ____ / ____

Today I am *Grateful* for _____

_____

_____

_____

_____

_____

Day: _____ *Date:* _____ / _____ / _____

Today I am *Grateful* for _____

_____

_____

_____

_____

_____

_____

Be not simply good - be good for something.
~ Henry David Thoreau

Day: _____ *Date:* _____ / _____ / _____

Today I am *Grateful* for _____

_____

_____

_____

_____

_____

_____

Day: _____ *Date:* ____ / ____ / ____

Today I am *Grateful* for _____

_____

_____

_____

_____

_____

In character, in manner, in style, in all things, the supreme
excellence is simplicity. ~ *Henry Wadsworth Longfellow*

Day: _____ *Date:* ____ / ____ / ____

Today I am *Grateful* for _____

_____

_____

_____

_____

_____

Day: _____ *Date:* ____ / ____ / ____

Today I am *Grateful* for _____

_____

_____

_____

_____

_____

You and I do not see things as they are. We see things as we are.
~ *Henry Ward Beecher*

Day: _____ *Date:* ____ / ____ / ____

Today I am *Grateful* for _____

_____

_____

_____

_____

_____

Day: _____ *Date:* ___ / ___ / ___

Today I am *Grateful* for _____

_____

_____

_____

_____

_____

The best thing one can do when it's raining is to let it rain.
~ *Henry Wadsworth Longfellow*

Day: _____ *Date:* ___ / ___ / ___

Today I am *Grateful* for _____

_____

_____

_____

_____

_____

Day: _____ *Date:* _____ / _____ / _____

Today I am *Grateful* for _____

_____

_____

_____

_____

_____

The sun does not shine for a few trees and flowers, but for the
wide world's joy. ~ *Henry Ward Beecher*

Day: _____ *Date:* _____ / _____ / _____

Today I am *Grateful* for _____

_____

_____

_____

_____

_____

Day: _____ *Date:* ____ / ____ / ____

Today I am *Grateful* for _____

_____

_____

_____

_____

_____

A picture is a poem without words.
~ *Horace*

Day: _____ *Date:* ____ / ____ / ____

Today I am *Grateful* for _____

_____

_____

_____

_____

_____

Day: _____ *Date:* ____ / ____ / ____

Today I am *Grateful* for _____

_____

_____

_____

_____

_____

_____

Tears of joy are like the summer rain drops pierced by sunbeams.
~ *Hosea Ballou*

Day: _____ *Date:* ____ / ____ / ____

Today I am *Grateful* for _____

_____

_____

_____

_____

_____

_____

Day: _____ *Date:* ___/___/___

Today I am *Grateful* for _____

_____

_____

_____

_____

_____

Happiness is not an ideal of reason, but of imagination.
~ Immanuel Kant

Day: _____ *Date:* ___/___/___

Today I am *Grateful* for _____

_____

_____

_____

_____

_____

Day: _____ *Date:* _____ / _____ / _____

Today I am *Grateful* for _____

_____

_____

_____

_____

_____

_____

It is beyond a doubt that all our knowledge begins with experience.
~ *Immanuel Kant*

Day: _____ *Date:* _____ / _____ / _____

Today I am *Grateful* for _____

_____

_____

_____

_____

_____

_____

Day: _____ *Date:* ____ / ____ / ____

Today I am *Grateful* for _____

_____

_____

_____

_____

_____

To every action there is always opposed an equal reaction.
~ *Isaac Newton*

Day: _____ *Date:* ____ / ____ / ____

Today I am *Grateful* for _____

_____

_____

_____

_____

_____

Day: _____ *Date:* ____ / ____ / ____

Today I am *Grateful* for _____

_____

_____

_____

_____

_____

Creativity is not the finding of a thing, but the making
something out of it after it is found. ~ *James Russell Lowell*

Day: _____ *Date:* ____ / ____ / ____

Today I am *Grateful* for _____

_____

_____

_____

_____

_____

Day: _____ *Date:* _____ / _____ / _____

Today I am *Grateful* for _____

_____

_____

_____

_____

_____

_____

Our will is always for our own good, but we do not always
see what that is. ~ *Jean-Jacques Rousseau*

Day: _____ *Date:* _____ / _____ / _____

Today I am *Grateful* for _____

_____

_____

_____

_____

_____

_____

Draw something

Day: _____ *Date:* ___ / ___ / ___

Today I am *Grateful* for _____

_____

_____

_____

_____

_____

The soul that sees beauty may sometimes walk alone.
~ *Johann Wolfgang von Goethe*

Day: _____ *Date:* ___ / ___ / ___

Today I am *Grateful* for _____

_____

_____

_____

_____

_____

Day: _____ *Date:* _____ / _____ / _____

Today I am *Grateful* for _____

_____

_____

_____

_____

_____

_____

Pleasure is none, if not diversified.
~ *John Donne*

Day: _____ *Date:* _____ / _____ / _____

Today I am *Grateful* for _____

_____

_____

_____

_____

_____

_____

Day: _____ *Date:* _____ / _____ / _____

Today I am *Grateful* for _____

_____

_____

_____

_____

_____

Nothing ever becomes real till it is experienced.
~ *John Keats*

Day: _____ *Date:* _____ / _____ / _____

Today I am *Grateful* for _____

_____

_____

_____

_____

_____

Day: _____ *Date:* ___/___/___

Today I am *Grateful* for _____

_____

_____

_____

_____

_____

What worries you, masters you.
~ *John Locke*

Day: _____ *Date:* ___/___/___

Today I am *Grateful* for _____

_____

_____

_____

_____

_____

Day: _____ *Date:* ____ / ____ / ____

Today I am *Grateful* for _____

_____

_____

_____

_____

_____

How glorious a greeting the sun gives the mountains!
~ John Muir

Day: _____ *Date:* ____ / ____ / ____

Today I am *Grateful* for _____

_____

_____

_____

_____

_____

Day: _____ *Date:* _____ / _____ / _____

Today I am *Grateful* for _____

_____

_____

_____

_____

_____

Three grand essentials to happiness in this life are something to do,
something to love, and something to hope for. ~ *Joseph Addison*

Day: _____ *Date:* _____ / _____ / _____

Today I am *Grateful* for _____

_____

_____

_____

_____

_____

Day: _____ *Date:* ____/____/____

Today I am *Grateful* for _____

_____

_____

_____

_____

_____

_____

In every walk with nature one receives far more than he seeks.
~ *John Muir*

Day: _____ *Date:* ____/____/____

Today I am *Grateful* for _____

_____

_____

_____

_____

_____

Day: _____ *Date:* _____ / _____ / _____

Today I am *Grateful* for _____

_____

_____

_____

_____

_____

Imagination is the eye of the soul.
~ *Joseph Joubert*

Day: _____ *Date:* _____ / _____ / _____

Today I am *Grateful* for _____

_____

_____

_____

_____

_____

Day: _____ *Date:* ____/____/____

Today I am *Grateful* for _____

_____

_____

_____

_____

_____

When unhappy, one doubts everything; when happy, one
doubts nothing. ~ *Joseph Roux*

Day: _____ *Date:* ____/____/____

Today I am *Grateful* for _____

_____

_____

_____

_____

_____

Day: _____ *Date:* ____ / ____ / ____

Today I am *Grateful* for _____

_____

_____

_____

_____

_____

There are lots of people who mistake their imagination for
their memory. ~ *Josh Billings*

Day: _____ *Date:* ____ / ____ / ____

Today I am *Grateful* for _____

_____

_____

_____

_____

_____

Day: _____ *Date:* ____ / ____ / ____

Today I am *Grateful* for _____

_____

_____

_____

_____

_____

When I let go of what I am, I become what I might be.
~ *Lao Tzu*

Day: _____ *Date:* ____ / ____ / ____

Today I am *Grateful* for _____

_____

_____

_____

_____

_____

Day: _____ *Date:* _____ / _____ / _____

Today I am *Grateful* for _____

_____

_____

_____

_____

_____

The risk of a wrong decision is preferable to the terror
of indecision. ~ *Maimonides*

Day: _____ *Date:* _____ / _____ / _____

Today I am *Grateful* for _____

_____

_____

_____

_____

_____

Day: _____ *Date:* ____/____/____

Today I am *Grateful* for _____

_____

_____

_____

_____

_____

The real voyage of discovery consists not in seeking new
landscapes, but in having new eyes. ~ *Marcel Proust*

Day: _____ *Date:* ____/____/____

Today I am *Grateful* for _____

_____

_____

_____

_____

_____

Day: _____ *Date:* _____ / _____ / _____

Today I am *Grateful* for _____

_____

_____

_____

_____

_____

Everything that happens happens as it should, and if you
observe carefully, you will find this to be so. ~ *Marcus Aurelius*

Day: _____ *Date:* _____ / _____ / _____

Today I am *Grateful* for _____

_____

_____

_____

_____

_____

Draw something

Day: _____ *Date:* ____/____/____

Today I am *Grateful* for _____

_____

_____

_____

_____

_____

_____

The pursuit, even of the best things, ought to be calm and tranquil.
~ *Marcus Tullius Cicero*

Day: _____ *Date:* ____/____/____

Today I am *Grateful* for _____

_____

_____

_____

_____

_____

_____

Day: _____ *Date:* ____ / ____ / ____

Today I am *Grateful* for _____

_____

_____

_____

_____

_____

Our life is what our thoughts make it.
~ *Marcus Aurelius*

Day: _____ *Date:* ____ / ____ / ____

Today I am *Grateful* for _____

_____

_____

_____

_____

_____

Day: _____ *Date:* ____ / ____ / ____

Today I am *Grateful* for _____

_____

_____

_____

_____

_____

Saying and doing are two things.
~ Matthew Henry

Day: _____ *Date:* ____ / ____ / ____

Today I am *Grateful* for _____

_____

_____

_____

_____

_____

Day: _____ *Date:* _____ / _____ / _____

Today I am *Grateful* for _____

_____

_____

_____

_____

_____

Rejoice in the things that are present; all else is beyond thee.
~ *Michel de Montaigne*

Day: _____ *Date:* _____ / _____ / _____

Today I am *Grateful* for _____

_____

_____

_____

_____

_____

Day: _____ *Date:* _____ / _____ / _____

Today I am *Grateful* for _____

_____

_____

_____

_____

_____

Tenderness is a virtue.
~ *Oliver Goldsmith*

Day: _____ *Date:* _____ / _____ / _____

Today I am *Grateful* for _____

_____

_____

_____

_____

_____

Day: _____ *Date:* ____/____/____

Today I am *Grateful* for _____

_____

_____

_____

_____

_____

_____

Keep love in your heart. A life without it is like a sunless garden
when the flowers are dead. ~ *Oscar Wilde*

Day: _____ *Date:* ____/____/____

Today I am *Grateful* for _____

_____

_____

_____

_____

_____

_____

Day: _____ *Date:* ____ / ____ / ____

Today I am *Grateful* for _____

_____

_____

_____

_____

_____

_____

Painting from nature is not copying the object; it is realizing one's
sensations. ~ *Paul Cezanne*

Day: _____ *Date:* ____ / ____ / ____

Today I am *Grateful* for _____

_____

_____

_____

_____

_____

Day: _____ *Date:* _____ / _____ / _____

Today I am *Grateful* for _____

_____

_____

_____

_____

_____

_____

Out of nothing can come, and nothing can become nothing.
~ *Persius*

Day: _____ *Date:* _____ / _____ / _____

Today I am *Grateful* for _____

_____

_____

_____

_____

_____

_____

Day: _____ *Date:* _____ / _____ / _____

Today I am *Grateful* for _____

_____

_____

_____

_____

_____

It is great happiness to be praised of them who are most praiseworthy.
~ *Philip Sidney*

Day: _____ *Date:* _____ / _____ / _____

Today I am *Grateful* for _____

_____

_____

_____

_____

_____

Day: _____ *Date:* _____ / _____ / _____

Today I am *Grateful* for _____

_____

_____

_____

_____

_____

Good actions give strength to ourselves and inspire good
actions in others. ~ *Plato*

Day: _____ *Date:* _____ / _____ / _____

Today I am *Grateful* for _____

_____

_____

_____

_____

_____

Day: _____ *Date:* _____ / _____ / _____

Today I am *Grateful* for _____

_____

_____

_____

_____

_____

When the mind is thinking it is talking to itself.
~ *Plato*

Day: _____ *Date:* _____ / _____ / _____

Today I am *Grateful* for _____

_____

_____

_____

_____

_____

Day: _____ *Date:* _____ / _____ / _____

Today I am *Grateful* for _____

_____

_____

_____

_____

_____

_____

Write it on your heart that every day is the best day in the year.
~ *Ralph Waldo Emerson*

Day: _____ *Date:* _____ / _____ / _____

Today I am *Grateful* for _____

_____

_____

_____

_____

_____

Day: _____ *Date:* ____/____/____

Today I am *Grateful* for _____

_____

_____

_____

_____

_____

That man is a success who has lived well, laughed often and
loved much. ~ *Robert Louis Stevenson*

Day: _____ *Date:* ____/____/____

Today I am *Grateful* for _____

_____

_____

_____

_____

_____

Day: _____ *Date:* ____ / ____ / ____

Today I am *Grateful* for _____

_____

_____

_____

_____

_____

_____

You cannot do a kindness too soon, for you never know how
soon it will be too late. ~ *Ralph Waldo Emerson*

Day: _____ *Date:* ____ / ____ / ____

Today I am *Grateful* for _____

_____

_____

_____

_____

_____

_____

Draw something

Day: _____ *Date:* _____ / _____ / _____

Today I am *Grateful* for _____

_____

_____

_____

_____

_____

_____

To forget oneself is to be happy.
~ *Robert Louis Stevenson*

Day: _____ *Date:* _____ / _____ / _____

Today I am *Grateful* for _____

_____

_____

_____

_____

_____

_____

Day: _____ *Date:* ____ / ____ / ____

Today I am *Grateful* for _____

_____

_____

_____

_____

_____

By experience we find out a short way by a long wandering.
~ *Roger Ascham*

Day: _____ *Date:* ____ / ____ / ____

Today I am *Grateful* for _____

_____

_____

_____

_____

_____

Day: _____ *Date:* _____ / _____ / _____

Today I am *Grateful* for _____

_____

_____

_____

_____

_____

Beauty surrounds us, but usually we need to be walking in
a garden to know it. ~ *Rumi*

Day: _____ *Date:* _____ / _____ / _____

Today I am *Grateful* for _____

_____

_____

_____

_____

_____

Day: _____ *Date:* _____ / _____ / _____

Today I am *Grateful* for _____

_____

_____

_____

_____

_____

Let the beauty of what you love be what you do.
~ *Rumi*

Day: _____ *Date:* _____ / _____ / _____

Today I am *Grateful* for _____

_____

_____

_____

_____

_____

Day: _____ *Date:* ____/____/____

Today I am *Grateful* for _____

_____

_____

_____

_____

_____

_____

To seek the highest good is to live well.
~ *Saint Augustine*

Day: _____ *Date:* ____/____/____

Today I am *Grateful* for _____

_____

_____

_____

_____

_____

_____

Day: _____ *Date:* _____ / _____ / _____

Today I am *Grateful* for _____

_____

_____

_____

_____

_____

Great works are performed not by strength but by perseverance.
~ *Samuel Johnson*

Day: _____ *Date:* _____ / _____ / _____

Today I am *Grateful* for _____

_____

_____

_____

_____

_____

Day: _____ *Date:* ____ / ____ / ____

Today I am *Grateful* for _____

_____

_____

_____

_____

_____

Wisdom begins in wonder.
~ Socrates

Day: _____ *Date:* ____ / ____ / ____

Today I am *Grateful* for _____

_____

_____

_____

_____

_____

Day: _____ *Date:* _____ / _____ / _____

Today I am *Grateful* for _____

_____

_____

_____

_____

_____

Success is dependent on effort.
~ *Sophocles*

Day: _____ *Date:* _____ / _____ / _____

Today I am *Grateful* for _____

_____

_____

_____

_____

_____

Day: _____ *Date:* _____ / _____ / _____

Today I am *Grateful* for _____

_____

_____

_____

_____

_____

Be as you wish to seem.
~ *Socrates*

Day: _____ *Date:* _____ / _____ / _____

Today I am *Grateful* for _____

_____

_____

_____

_____

_____

Day: _____ *Date:* ____ / ____ / ____

Today I am *Grateful* for _____

_____

_____

_____

_____

_____

Our happiness depends on wisdom all the way.
~ Sophocles

Day: _____ *Date:* ____ / ____ / ____

Today I am *Grateful* for _____

_____

_____

_____

_____

Day: _____ *Date:* ____ / ____ / ____

Today I am *Grateful* for _____

_____

_____

_____

_____

_____

_____

The best thinking has been done in solitude. The worst has
been done in turmoil. ~ *Thomas A. Edison*

Day: _____ *Date:* ____ / ____ / ____

Today I am *Grateful* for _____

_____

_____

_____

_____

_____

_____

Day: _____ *Date:* _____ / _____ / _____

Today I am *Grateful* for _____

_____

_____

_____

_____

_____

The things that we love tell us what we are.
~ *Thomas Aquinas*

Day: _____ *Date:* _____ / _____ / _____

Today I am *Grateful* for _____

_____

_____

_____

_____

_____

Day: _____ *Date:* _____ / _____ / _____

Today I am *Grateful* for _____

_____

_____

_____

_____

_____

Our greatest weakness lies in giving up. The most certain way to
succeed is always to try just one more time. ~ *Thomas A. Edison*

Day: _____ *Date:* _____ / _____ / _____

Today I am *Grateful* for _____

_____

_____

_____

_____

_____

Day: _____ *Date:* ____ / ____ / ____

Today I am *Grateful* for _____

_____

_____

_____

_____

_____

Wonder is the desire for knowledge.
~ *Thomas Aquinas*

Day: _____ *Date:* ____ / ____ / ____

Today I am *Grateful* for _____

_____

_____

_____

_____

_____

Draw something

Day: _____ *Date:* _____ / _____ / _____

Today I am *Grateful* for _____

_____

_____

_____

_____

_____

_____

It is the heart always that sees, before the head can see.
~ *Thomas Carlyle*

Day: _____ *Date:* _____ / _____ / _____

Today I am *Grateful* for _____

_____

_____

_____

_____

_____

_____

Day: _____ *Date:* ____/____/____

Today I am *Grateful* for _____

_____

_____

_____

_____

_____

_____

Every noble work is at first impossible.
~ *Thomas Carlyle*

Day: _____ *Date:* ____/____/____

Today I am *Grateful* for _____

_____

_____

_____

_____

_____

_____

Day: _____ *Date:* _____ / _____ / _____

Today I am *Grateful* for _____

_____

_____

_____

_____

_____

_____

If it were not for hopes, the heart would break.
~ Thomas Fuller

Day: _____ *Date:* _____ / _____ / _____

Today I am *Grateful* for _____

_____

_____

_____

_____

_____

Day: _____ *Date:* ____/____/____

Today I am *Grateful* for _____

_____

_____

_____

_____

_____

> The harder the conflict, the more glorious the triumph.
> ~ *Thomas Paine*

Day: _____ *Date:* ____/____/____

Today I am *Grateful* for _____

_____

_____

_____

_____

_____

Day: _____ *Date:* _____ / _____ / _____

Today I am *Grateful* for _____

_____

_____

_____

_____

_____

Life is the flower for which love is the honey.
~ *Victor Hugo*

Day: _____ *Date:* _____ / _____ / _____

Today I am *Grateful* for _____

_____

_____

_____

_____

_____

Day: _____ *Date:* _____ / _____ / _____

Today I am *Grateful* for _____

_____

_____

_____

_____

_____

The way to know life is to love many things.
~ *Vincent Van Gogh*

Day: _____ *Date:* _____ / _____ / _____

Today I am *Grateful* for _____

_____

_____

_____

_____

_____

Day: _____ *Date:* _____ / _____ / _____

Today I am *Grateful* for _____

_____

_____

_____

_____

_____

Persevere and preserve yourselves for better circumstances.
~ *Virgil*

Day: _____ *Date:* _____ / _____ / _____

Today I am *Grateful* for _____

_____

_____

_____

_____

_____

Day: _____ *Date:* ____ / ____ / ____

Today I am *Grateful* for _____

_____

_____

_____

_____

_____

By appreciation, we make excellence in others our own property.
~ *Voltaire*

Day: _____ *Date:* ____ / ____ / ____

Today I am *Grateful* for _____

_____

_____

_____

_____

_____

Day: _____ *Date:* _____ / _____ / _____

Today I am *Grateful* for _____

_____

_____

_____

_____

_____

Keep your face always toward the sunshine - and shadows
will fall behind you. ~ *Walt Whitman*

Day: _____ *Date:* _____ / _____ / _____

Today I am *Grateful* for _____

_____

_____

_____

_____

_____

Day: _____ *Date:* _____ / _____ / _____

Today I am *Grateful* for _____

_____

_____

_____

_____

_____

_____

You never know what is enough unless you know what is
more than enough. ~ *William Blake*

Day: _____ *Date:* _____ / _____ / _____

Today I am *Grateful* for _____

_____

_____

_____

_____

_____

Day: _____ *Date:* _____ / _____ / _____

Today I am *Grateful* for _____

_____

_____

_____

_____

_____

A gentle word, a kind look, a good-natured smile can work
wonders and accomplish miracles. ~ *William Hazlitt*

Day: _____ *Date:* _____ / _____ / _____

Today I am *Grateful* for _____

_____

_____

_____

_____

_____

Day: _____ *Date:* _____ / _____ / _____

Today I am *Grateful* for _____

_____

_____

_____

_____

_____

The greatest weapon against stress is our ability to choose
one thought over another. ~ *William James*

Day: _____ *Date:* _____ / _____ / _____

Today I am *Grateful* for _____

_____

_____

_____

_____

_____

Day: _____ *Date:* _____ / _____ / _____

Today I am *Grateful* for _____

_____

_____

_____

_____

_____

We are here to add what we can to life, not to get what we
can from life. ~ *William Osler*

Day: _____ *Date:* _____ / _____ / _____

Today I am *Grateful* for _____

_____

_____

_____

_____

_____

Day: _____ *Date:* _____ / _____ / _____

Today I am *Grateful* for _____

_____

_____

_____

_____

_____

_____

To begin, begin.
~ *William Wordsworth*

Day: _____ *Date:* _____ / _____ / _____

Today I am *Grateful* for _____

_____

_____

_____

_____

_____

Draw something

Notes

Notes

Printed in the USA
CPSIA information can be obtained
at www.ICGtesting.com
LVHW021110281223
767380LV00077B/83